I0441878

ANTI VIRUS, COMBATING AND PROTECTING AGAINST COVID 19 VIRUS THROUGH GOODAIRE SANZ

BY

RICHARD YECK
INVENTOR AND FOUNDER OF GOODAIRE PTE LTD

ASSISTED BY

SUCHITTHRA VASU
LLB HONS LONDON
LLM MONASH MELBOURNE
LAWYER/WRITER/AUTHOR AND NOVELIST

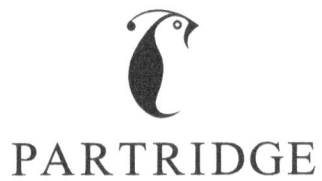

PARTRIDGE

To order additional copies of this book, contact
Toll Free 800 101 2657 (Singapore)
Toll Free 1 800 81 7340 (Malaysia)
orders.singapore@partridgepublishing.com

www.partridgepublishing.com/singapore

CONTENTS

DEDICATION

Dedicated to my beloved parents in heaven, to my loving wife Bellice Teo my two lovely daughters, Julia Yeck and Bernice Yeck who have stood by me like the Rock of Gibraltar and given me overwhelming strength. Last but not least to the cause of uplifting mankind from suffering.

ACKNOWLEDGEMENTS

I wish to thank the following persons who have helped me in my career or in my life one way or another, in alphabetical order

Chia Chong Wan
Chua Chun Guan, Christopher
Hu Yi Gang
Lee Chee Seng, Chris

Lim Kwang Kiat
Lim Charlie
Ong Beng Leong, Michael
See Lub Hwee
Tan Seng Kim (late)
Toh Siew In (Ms)
Tan Soo Hwang, Dickson
Tan Soo Yam, Eric
Tan Swee Lin, Lyn (Ms)
Tan Puay Tong
Teo Thian Chye, Stanley
Wong Yoke Meng (Dr)
Wu Yuan Cheng
Yek Wei Ming, Albert
Yek Christopher
Yeo Bee Choon Jeffrey
Yet Allan
Zheng Wei
Adanan Cherus

Joshua Kwame Ahalivor
Apostle Anthony Kwabla Ahalivor
David Pierra, Professor
Zairi Jaal, Professor
Zhan Juan Juan
Zheng wei
Last but not least,
Ms Suchitthra Vasu
Dr Patrick Fernandez and
Mr Chang Hee Kuan for the production of this book

PREFACE

Every now and then, some great person screams "Eureka" inventing something special and unusual for the advancement and the better quality of life. For example, Bill Gates, for his innovations in the highly advance state of technology we are in today. The Wright brothers for inventing aircrafts so that we can cross the big oceans and bring us to lands afar. The list can go on and on. The one thing about life and its inherent feature is change and change is constant. Life is uncertain and the only thing that is certain is death which eventuates for every human being. Still, despite these tremendous feats and accolades there is one thing that appears not within our control. This is when the world is afflicted with sickness stemming from various viruses. No one knows if this is man made or an act of mother nature or an act of God but whatever the term used these deadly viruses can topple the world over, causing immense global disaster to the health and well being of humanity, leave alone the economic catastrophe. Just when humanity thinks you have got it made and every thing is hunky dory and that this world is a beautiful place to live in, a disaster strikes and it has been the case from time immemorial. In the 14th Century 50 million people lost their lives to the plague known as the: Black Death:

If we look back at the track record, the world has seen situations of extreme difficulty and challenges over some of the 23 most deadly viruses.

Mankind has been combating viruses since before our species had even evolved into its modern form. For some viral diseases, with advancement in medical science, vaccines and antiviral drugs have developed to stop infections from spreading rampantly, and have made sick people recover. For example, smallpox —has been eradicated.

However, we are a long way from winning the battle against viruses. In recent years, several viruses have infected humans from animals and causing huge outbreaks, and causing a huge amount of deaths. For instance the 2014-2016 Ebola outbreak in West Africa killed up to 90% of the people it infected, making it the most lethal member of the Ebola family.

However, there are other viruses out there that are equally deadly, and some that are even deadlier. Some viruses, including the novel corona virus currently driving outbreaks around the globe, have lower fatality rates, but are still a serious threat to public health as we have yet found out the means to eradicate them. It appears the onus in still on humanity to find vaccines or other means to combat and protect ourselves from these deadly viruses.

This book is a small book but with a serious intent. It takes a journey on a birds eye view on some of the deadliest viruses afflicting mankind on this planet and will narrow down to the current day Corona Virus that has plagued the globe and which the WHO authorities have indicated as an enemy of humanity. In the current wake of things, it is incumbent to address methods of hygiene that one must. as a mandatory obligation to humanity at large, adopt methods to safeguard the spread of Corona Virus. This is so that things don't get exacerbated and out of control. Since the onus is on mankind to make this world a better place than we found it, there are scientific methods and medical methods to combat and protect humanity against these viruses such as adopting hygienic methods as a way of life so that the spread of infections can be curtailed. GoodAire, the company responsible for this book addresses the current situation of the catastrophic outbreak of Corona Virus globally and offers simple scientifically tested methods to combat the spread of this virus. GoodAire has done extensive research on this subject matter and offers some intelligent solutions that should be adopted and should be addressed with all seriousness. Before we delve in the constructive propositions that GOOD AIRE has to offer, let us take a journey into some of the deadliest viruses that have affected humanity and planet earth and get on to being updated with Coronavirus. Coronavirus today is a universal problem and an ongoing one and no one has found the medical option or vaccine to eradicate it. The virus causes unspeakable suffering and has resulted in hundreds and thousands of deaths. There is also the pain, despair and anguish of loosing loved ones as it takes away old and young and it has been said it has no passport as it is a global pandemic. As of the writing of this book 17 April 2020 there are

Coronavirus Cases:
2,165,586
Deaths:
144,341
Recovered:
546,269

Here is a bird's eye view of the content of this book. Now, we will journey into the history of the deadliest viruses that have attacked humanity then focus on the current Corona Virus and then expand on the scientific well researched solutions GoodAire Sanz has to offer in combating and protecting against deadly viruses which includes Corona Virus. This virus has caused havoc permeating into the fabric of society and destroying lifestyles. It destroys the freedom of movement of humanity across the oceans where flights are grounded and freedom of movement even on a domestic level. It destroys one's health one's well being and destroys life itself bringing complete devastation. What an ungodly, sinister affair, surely this was not how mother nature meant it for humanity yet where did it stem from.? It is also known as the Wuhan virus believed to originate from the Wuhan province of China. It is probably not politically correct to use the word 'Wuhan' virus. The latest finding suggests three strains of this SARS-CoV-2 virus.

Researchers from Cambridge, UK, and Germany have reconstructed the early 'evolutionary paths' of SARS-CoV-2 in humans – as the infection spread from Wuhan out to Europe and North America – using genetic network techniques.'

The research revealed three distinct 'variants' of SARS-CoV-2, consisting of clusters of closely related lineages, which they label 'A', 'B' and 'C'. Versions of 'A' were seen in Chinese individuals, and Americans reported to have lived in Wuhan, and mutated versions of 'A' were found in patients from the USA and Australia. Wuhan's major virus type, 'B', was prevalent in patients from across East Asia. However, the variant didn't travel much beyond the region without further mutations – implying a 'founder event' in Wuhan, or 'resistance' against this type of coronavirus outside East Asia, say researchers. The 'C' variant is the major European type, found in early patients from France, Italy, Sweden and England. It is absent from the study's Chinese mainland sample but seen in Singapore, Hong Kong and South Korea.

Variant 'A', most closely related to the virus found in both bats and pangolins, is described as 'the root of the outbreak' by researchers. Type 'B' is derived from 'A', separated by two mutations, then 'C' is in turn a "daughter" of 'B'. These findings seem to support the latest separate reports in USA and Europe where Covid-19 was found much earlier than the first reported case in Wuhan, China.

GoodAire Sanz through well researched studies and scientific methods offers practical solutions to purify the air surrounding us to combat this virus and also to bring back a higher level of hygiene. The basis of their theories is bent on combating and protecting one and all. Mr. Richard Yeck CEO of GoodAire brings out this book at this crucial time to create awareness to the international community at large with a view to apply time tested and scientific methods to combat, march on, protect and win the battle. It propagates the theory that it is not just about medical treatment it is also about adopting the highest standard of hygiene through air purifiers using masks and sanitizers that will keep the individual and atmosphere clean and wholesome so the virus cannot survive. We all have a part to play, an individual part to play in this battle so let GoodAire Sanz unlock some golden keys to the road to recovery.

CHAPTER 1

VIRUSES AND THE HISTORY OF PANDEMICS

What Is a Virus?

Only and only if you know how harmful a virus is, will it hit home the hard fact that you need to protect against catching a virus And, there are some well researched methods on how to protect yourself which you will read later on in this book. Also, the sad fact is there are viruses on this planet earth and there are dangers lurking in every nook and corner when they start multiplying and replicating themselves in the host body. A virus is a microscopic agent that can only replicate or remain alive in a living organism be it a human, animal or plant and then it can replicate itself and multiply changing the cells of the host body.

A virus is a potent substance which is within an organic particle. It attacks living cells and goes through a metabolic process to reproduce and in the end creates a new wave of viral particles.

How this happens varies. At times, they can go through an incubation period, develop their genetic material into this host DNA and then after the waiting period it can create more and new viruses. Lytic Cycle is the term given to viruses that explode and expand in numbers and reproduce rapidly. In a human body this has an adverse effect on the health of the individual needless to say. In sum total, viruses are dangerous and can cause illnesses that can be very harmful. When invaded by a virus if not medically treated as soon as the symptoms occurs, it can lead to causalities depending on how lethal the virus is. So, symptoms making a person feel unwell should not be ignored and should be attended to immediately with proper medical attention to avoid the condition of the individual exacerbating and sometimes even leading to death. For most viral infections, medical treatments can only help with symptoms while you wait for your immune system to fight off the virus. Antibiotics do not work for viral infections.

Occurrences like influenza, are a viral infection, we treat the symptoms like cough and cold, and once the usual green phlegm is produced, it is a bacterial infection, and can thus be treated with the usual antibiotics.

In the context of the current Covid-19 pandemic, in the rapid antibody test kits, this is what we are looking for ie the presence of IgM and IgG antibodies, which show our body has started to "fight" back. Getting viral infections is part and parcel of daily living, we cannot avoid it because there are numerous viruses that we are exposed to. In reality, whether we succumb to it in a serious way, is largely dependent on our immune system.

SIZE OF VIRUSES

Virus comes from a Latin word meaning poisonous liquids. The virus sizes vary from as tiny as - 17 nanometre wide Porcine Circovirus, for example - to huge monstrous sizes that pose as a challenge to the very definition of the word 'virus', such as the 2.3 micrometre Tupanvirus.

Their constitution can be very complicated being made of, differing proteins or made up of a multitude of shells and envelopes to accelerate their infection and reproduction.

Viruses can be encoded in a multitude of ways. The basis of Rotaviruses are on a double strand of RNA, for example. Corona viruses have a single strand of RNA, which is a 'positive sense'. This is because it can be developed into new proteins. Influenza for instance has a negative sense RNA, which means it requires a further transcribing step prior to making proteins.

Smallpox and herpes viruses are DNA viruses, which on entry push the host to transcribe its genome into RNA.

Genomes sizes also differ. The largest ones can be over a million base pairs long. On an antithesis, an RNA virus that infects bacteria, called MS2, has merely 3,500 base pairs.

It is not known how many types of viruses thrive in this world, The sad fact is numbers are climbing. Still researchers are subscribing to new methods to elicit for classified and unfamiliar genetic signatures in the soil, oceans, and also the skies. Lo and behold it appears that a rough estimate is that there could be as a huge amount as 100 million types of virus loitering like rogues on the surface of the earth. We are all vulnerable and can fall prey to catching a virus infection and if it spreads before you know it, a pandemic can unwittingly erupt.

Virus Alive?

A question that has plagued the minds of scientists over the years is whether viruses are alive. The ecological system of the world has changed and it is suggested under the new school of thought is that viruses are considered to be part and parcel of our complex living form and it circulates amongst all living organisms. It is believed that "Virions" are considered dormant particles that exist in the environment but they come alive and become active once they become part of a cell. They then in turn become alive with a characteristic of their own by borrowing the biochemistry of the host and then multiply. As such, they are a blend of chemistry and biology and thereby there is no clear demarcation into the living and non living.

What is a Pandemic?

A pandemic is the global outbreak of a disease. There have existed many examples in history, the most recent being the COVID-19 pandemic, declared as such by the World Health Organization on March 12, 2020.

THE BLACK DEATH

All hell broke loose. This was one of the worst pandemics in history. The Black Death was a tragic global disaster of an epidemic of bubonic plague that struck Europe and Asia in the mid-1300s. It was a terrifying experience for the world indeed. This was perhaps the most wretched, cursed and macabre period in world history for the plight of humanity. It has been said by Ole J. Benedictow that the **Black Death killed** 50 million **people** in the 14th century, or 60 per cent of Europe's entire population. The disastrous mortal disease known as the **Black Death** permeated through Europe in the years 1346-53. And it lingered on for quite some while too.

The Start of the Plague

The plague arrived from Europe in October 1347, when 12 ships from the Black Sea docked at the Sicilian port of Messina. People who came to the docks were met with a rude shock. Most sailors on board the ships were dead, and those still alive were seriously ill. They were covered with black boils that had blood and pus coming out of them. The Sicilian authorities rapidly instructed the fleet of "death ships" out of the harbor, but it was too late: The next five years, the Black Death killed more than 20 million people in Europe being one-third of the continent's population.

Even before the ships full of deceased sailors embarked into port at Messina, many Europeans had heard about a "Great Pestilence" that was setting the stage for a deadly path on the trade routes of the Near and Far East. The disease permeated and gravely affected the people on these trade routes in the early 1340s, affecting China, India, Persia, Syria and Egypt.

This horrendous and sinister plague is believed to have its origins in Asia over 2,000 years ago and was spread by trading ships. However, there are other theories that indicated the plague, the progenitor, of the Black Death may have existed in Europe as early as 3000 B.C.

Symptoms of Plague

To describe the horror of those afflicted" the Italian poet Giovanni Boccaccio wrote, "at the beginning of the malady, certain swellings, either on the groin or under the armpits...waxed to the bigness of a common apple, others to the size of an egg, some more and some less, and these the vulgar named plague-boils." No one was prepared for this at all. The Bubonic Plague invaded the lymphatic system, resulting in the swelling of the lymph nodes. The infection could spread to the blood or lungs if left untreated. The chilling reality of the cold-blooded symptoms of Bubonic Plague were fever, chills, vomiting, diarrhea, terrible aches and pains—and finally death. It took the world by a rude shock with a bitter ending for those afflicted. It was frighteningly infectious so that it could spread just by touching the afflicted person's clothes. It was so robust at harming people that one could be perfectly well at bedtime and wake up dead by the morning.

Comprehending the Plague

Currently, scientists are of the view that the Black Death, known as the plague, is spread by a bacillus a germ called *Yersina pestis* discovered by the French biologist Alexandre Yersin at the end of the 19th century.

They now have discovered that the bacillus spreads from person to person through the air, as well as through the bite of infected fleas and rats. These pests could be found almost everywhere in medieval Europe, but they were particularly rampant aboard ships of all kinds. This is how the contagious plague spread from one European port city to another.

It was not very long after it struck Messina, the Black Death spread to the port of Marseilles in France and the port of Tunis in North Africa. It then made its way to Rome and Florence, which were the center of trade routes. And then, by the middle of 1348, it affected Paris, Bordeaux, Lyon and London.

At that time, this bleak, doom and gloom sequence of events could not all be comprehended. There was no logical explanation for this and no one had any knowledge how exactly the Black Death spread from one patient to another. Still worse, there was a dearth of information on how to prevent it and be protected from it

TREATMENT OF PLAGUE

At that time when medical science was not developed and physicians relied on raw techniques such as bloodletting and boil-lancing (

. These practices proved too dangerous as well as unsanitary exacerbating the conditions of life. Also, some adopted superstitious practices like burning aromatic herbs and bathing in rosewater or vinegar.

There was panic every where. Healthy people avoided the sick. Doctors did not attend to patients; priests did administer last rites; and shopkeepers closed their stores. There was an exodus of people from the cities fleeing to the countryside, but neither that was a safe option as they could not escape the disease: It affected animals as well such as cows, sheep, goats, pigs and chickens.

People, desperate to save themselves, abandoned their sick and dying loved ones. It was indeed a very sorry state of affairs. The very fabric of society and communal living in harmony had disintegrated and humanity was progressively being destroyed with venom that seemingly saw no abatement.

BLACK DEATH- WAS IT RETRIBUTION?

People could not comprehend the biology of the disease, so they were of the belief that the Black Death was divine punishment and retribution for sins against God. It appeared to them that, the only way to overcome the plague was to win God's forgiveness. Some people believed that the way to do this was to purge their communities of heretics and other troublemakers, so many thousands of Jews were massacred in 1348 and 1349. and this led to many fleeing the regions of Eastern Europe to find a safe habitat for fear of the raging mobs in the cities:

Social Distancing and Quarantine in Medieval Times to Fight the Black Death?

The plague lingered on and returned revengefully years later. However, officials in the Venetian-controlled port city of Ragusa curtailed its spread where sailors were kept in isolation; until they got the green signal that they were not carrying the disease. They created social distancing that relied on isolation to slow the spread of the disease. So, this concept of social distancing and quarantine had its roots embedded in history as far back as the medieval times

The sailors were kept on their ships for 30 days (a *trentino*). The period later increased to 40 days, or a *quarantine*—This practice is still used today.

Does Plague Still Exist?

The Black Death epidemic had run its course by the early 1350s. However the plague resurfaced every few generations for centuries. Since sanitation and public-health practices have since been enhanced it has greatly cushioned the impact of the disease but it is not completely eliminated Modern medication such as antibiotics are available and can treat the plague but, according to The World Health Organization, today there are still about 1,000 to 3,000 cases of plague lingering on per year.

A Historical Journey of 22 Worst Epidemics and Pandemics

The sad state of affairs and a blatant reality is life in itself is entirely fragile. There is no guarantee of a good life once you come into this world though there are moments of joy and goodness too. As we go down history one realizes that epidemics and global pandemics have savagely robbed humanity of health and dignity of life throughout, more often than not causing a mutation in the course of history. What is it? Is it the wrath of God? Is it the change in the ecological system? Has this in turn caused destruction to humanity because humanity has abused Mother Nature? No one has the answer. Still as dumbfounded as we are, we have no choice but to fight for survival. Medical science with the most brilliant scientist's brains at work has over the years evolved, finding vaccines and medication to address these problems. This book points to the fact that medicines are not enough in the combat of deadly viruses one also needs to purify the air we breathe sanitize our hands and have a higher level of hygiene in our fight against these awful viruses that debilitates man's existence. GoodAire has provided some interesting, formidable and effective methods for combating viruses and for protection against them. We will delve into this in detail in the last chapter of this book to show you the latest innovations and the avenue for sound and effective protection. For now, let us journey to the battlefield and look at history and what we need to deal with. What is it that precipitates as these viruses ending in terrible suffering to one's health and well being? These viruses that invade the bodies of mankind causing absolute havoc and destroys one's health dates from prehistoric to modern times to today's wretched Corona virus

What is the difference between Epidemic and Pandemic

A disease can be declared an *epidemic* when it spreads over a wide area and many people are taken ill at the same time. If the spread exacerbates, an epidemic can become a *pandemic*, when it spread across the oceans and affects an even wider geographical area. As in the current case of Coronavirus it is a global pandemic as the parameters of the disease have traveled round the world and large and phenomenal proportions of people have become affected.

1. Prehistoric epidemic: China3000 B.C.

In China, 5,000 years ago, an epidemic completely devastated a village. The dead bodies were put together in a house which was later burned down. The epidemic did not spare any one. The old and young were reduced to skeletons which were found inside this house known as the archaeological site called "Hamin Mangha.". As the deaths happened suddenly and rapidly there was no time for proper burials. Also, a site called Miazigou in North East China in an around the same time in prehistoric times showed evidence of mass burial. These archaeological prehistoric sites are discoveries of an epidemic that destroyed the total regions

2. Plague of Athens: 430 B.C.

Around 430 B.C., after the war between Athens and Sparta began, an epidemic devastated the people of Athens for five years. About 100,000 people lost their lives. Suddenly people in good health experienced a sinister heat in their head's inflammation of the eyes, throat and tongues. The suffering was excruciatingly painful and sordid. No one could pin point what this disease was all about. Some school of thoughts was that it was typhoid and Ebola. Some said it was due to the consequences of over crowding due to the war. The war did not end till 404 BC when the epidemic slowly subsided

3. Antonine Plague: A.D. 165-180

The Antonine Plague began when soldiers came back to the Roman Empire after the war against Parthia It was small pox that killed over 5 million people. This was when Rome was at the pinnacle of its power. The Christian belief thrived during the period when the plague happened. There was civil war from barbarian groups during this period after A.D.180

4. Plague of Cyprian: A.D. 250-271

The Plague of Cyprian killed 5,000 people on a daily basis in Rome alone. Archaeologists in Luxor found a massive burial site where masses were plague victims. A thick layer of lime in those days was used as a disinfectant covered their bodies which were burnt in a giant bonfire. The Bishop of Carthage indicated that this was a signal that the end of the world was imminent

5. Plague of Justinian: A.D. 541-542

Bubonic Plague that occurred in the Byzantine Empire set the stage for its descent. 10% of the world population died and there was horrendous devastation

6. The Black Death: 1346-1353

The Black Death spread voraciously from Asia to Europe and destroyed more than half of Europe's population. It was due to a strain of bacterium Yersinia Pestis spread by fleas and infected rodents

7. Cocoliztli epidemic: 1545-1548

Cocoliztli epidemic was a viral hemorrhagic fever. It killed 15 million inhabitants of Mexico and Central America. Among a population already weakened by extreme drought, the disease proved to be utterly catastrophic. "Cocoliztli" is the Aztec word for "pest."

Recent research indicates that DNA from the skeletons of victims showed they were infected with a species of *Salmonella* known as *S. paratyphi C*, this causes enteric fever, a kind of fever which was typhoid. Symptoms of Enteric fever are high fever, dehydration and gastrointestinal problems. This is still a prevalent threat today.

8. American Plagues: 16th century

European explorers brought a cluster of Eurasian diseases to America called the American Plague. These illnesses, included smallpox which were the cause of the collapse of the Inca and Aztec civilizations. 90% of the population in the Western Hemisphere died from this disease.

9. Great Plague of London: 1665-1666

Due to The Black Death's major outbreak in Great Britain there was a large exodus from London, led by King Charles II. The plague began in April 1665 and spreading through the summer months. The spread was due to fleas from plague-infected rodents. It is estimated that when plague ended, about 100,000 people, died

10. Great Plague of Marseille: 1720-1723

The Great Plague of Marseille began when a ship called Grand-Saint-Antoine docked in Marseille; France. It carried cargo from the eastern Mediterranean. Despite the fact that the ship was quarantined, plague rapidly spread into the city, probably through fleas on plague-infected rodents. Plague spread rapidly, 30% of the population of Marseille were destroyed.

11. Russian plague: 1770-1772

The Plague in Moscow, caused terror of those quarantined where violence. erupted amongst disgruntled citizens. Riots became rampant through the city. When the plague ended, a total of 100,000 people is estimated to have died.

12. Philadelphia yellow fever epidemic: 1793

At this time, yellow fever spread in Philadelphia, the United States' capital. Officials were of the wrong view that slaves were immune so that people of African origin were recruited to care for the sick.

The disease is carried by mosquitoes, and there was a population boom during the hot humid summer season in Philadelphia that year. Only when winter arrived did the mosquitoes die. Then the epidemic came to an end. More than 5,000 people had died.

13. Flu pandemic: 1889-1890

In the modern industrial age, influenza viruses caused devastation. Within a few months, the disease spread round the globe. 1 million people perished. In just five weeks, the epidemic reached the apex of mortality.

Initial cases were in Russia. The virus spread rapidly throughout St. Petersburg before it spread throughout Europe and globally, even though air travel did not exist at that time

14. American polio epidemic: 1916

Polio epidemic rooted in New York City brought about 27,000 cases and 6,000 deaths in the United States. This disease mainly affects children and at times leaves survivors with permanent disabilities.

Polio epidemics existed in the United States until the Salk vaccine was developed in 1954. Since the vaccine became widely available, there was a drop in cases. The last reported polio case in the United States was in 1979. Worldwide vaccination efforts have been a cure for the disease, although it is not completely eradicated.

15. Spanish Flu: 1918-1920

500 million people from the South Seas to the North Pole became victims of Spanish Flu. The flu spread and due to the cramped conditions of soldiers and poor wartime nutrition that many people were experiencing during World War I. Though the name is Spanish Flu, the disease did not start in Spain Generally people erroneously believed the illness was specific to Spain.

16. Asian Flu: 1957-1958

The Asian Flu was another global pandemic for influenza. With its origins in China, 1 million lives perished the virus was caused by a blend of avian flu viruses.

It is interesting to note that according to the Centers for Disease Control and Prevention the disease spread rapidly and was reported in Singapore in February 1957, Hong Kong in April 1957, and the coastal cities of the United States in the summer of 1957. Worldwide death toll was more than 1.1 million worldwide, of which 116,000 deaths were in the United States.

17. AIDS pandemic and epidemic: 1981-present day

AIDS claimed an estimated 35 million lives since it surfaced. HIV, which is the virus that causes AIDS, believed to develop from a chimpanzee virus and transferred to humans in West Africa in the 1920s. The virus spread around the world. In late 20th Century AIDS was a pandemic. Records show 64% of 40 million living with <u>human immunodeficiency virus</u> (HIV) are on sub-Saharan Africa.

For years, the disease had no known cure. Now medication has since developed in the 1990s giving people a normal life span with proper medical treatment.

18 SARS (Severe Acute Respiratory Syndrome) 2002-2003

SARS coronavirus (SARS-CoV) – virus emerged in 2003. SARS-CoV is believed to be an animal virus, perhaps bats, that spread to other animals (civet cats) and first infected humans in the Guangdong province of southern China in 2002.

26 countries were affected by this epidemic which resulted in more than 8000 cases in 2003 The symptoms are influenza-like Persons affected suffer fever, malaise, myalgia, headache, diarrhea, and shivering (rigors) Countries/areas to which it spread from The Centers for Disease Control

and Prevention human-to-human were predominantly in Toronto in Canada, Hong Kong Special Administrative Region of China, Chinese Taipei, Singapore, and Hanoi in Viet Nam.

19. H1N1 Swine Flu pandemic: 2009-2010

In 2009 swine flu pandemic was caused by a new strain of H1N1. It had its origins in Mexico in the spring of 2009. From thereon, it spread to the rest of the world. Within a year, the virus infected 1.4 billion people globally. It killed between 151,700 and 575,400 people.

According to The Prevention, the 2009 flu pandemic mainly affected children and young adults, and 80% of the deaths were in people below 65. Interestingly, in the case of the swine flu, older people seemed to have enough immunity to the group of viruses that H1N1 belongs to were not affected. Now a vaccine for the H1N1 virus is included in the annual flu vaccine.

20. West African Ebola epidemic: 2014-2016

Ebola spread in West Africa between 2014 and 2016, There were 28,600 reported cases and 11,325 deaths. The first case was in Guinea in December 2013. It then spread rapidly to Liberia and Sierra Leone. Most of the cases and deaths happened in those three countries. A smaller number happened in Nigeria, Mali, Senegal, the United States and Europe.

Ebola, has no cure. There are however ongoing efforts to find a vaccine. Ebola originated in Sudan and the Democratic Republic of Congo in 1976, and the virus comes from bats.

21. Zika Virus epidemic: 2015-present day

The impact of Zika epidemic in South America and Central America is still uncertain. Scientists are doing their utmost to bring the virus under control. The Zika virus is spread through mosquitoes of the *Aedes* genu. There is a school of thought that it can be sexually transmitted in humans.

Though <u>Zika</u> is usually not harmful to adults or children, it can affect unborn infants in the womb resulting in birth defects. Mosquitoes carrying Zika flourish best in warm, humid climates, so that South America, Central America and parts of the southern United States including countries in the tropics are vulnerable to it.

22 Dengue The 2019–2020 dengue fever epidemic Present day

This is an infectious viral infection called Dengue fever. Particularly rampant in countries of Southeast Asia, being the Philippines, Malaysia, Vietnam, and Bangladesh,[1] Pakistan, Thailand, Singapore, and Laos. The cause of spread of the disease has been worsened by the unavailability of vaccination levels in some regions and, the growing population of mosquitoes. Mosquitoes are the main carriers of the disease Countries affected have ongoing methods of controlling the epidemic through vaccination efforts, and through other efforts to stop mosquito breeding.

Dengue fever is more prevalent in tropical and subtropical regions It is a spread by mosquitoes. It has dramatically surfaced as an epidemic of dengue in the tropics globally. A major public health concern is the life-threatening complication of the illness called dengue hemorrhagic fever

CHAPTER 2

CURRENT DAY GLOOM AND DOOM COVID 19 GLOBALLY

A killer bug, today, looms the earth causing terrible illness and claiming thousands of lives around the globe. This is a highly infectious disease and the outbreak has been in many countries worldwide. It is not at all discriminatory as it does not spare anyone It has spread and caused infections from heads of states to menial workers and covers all cross sections of society from young to old, rich or poor regardless of race. All men are equal in the eyes of this killer bug and it is rapidly spreading. Governments around the world have lost control though they have implemented safe distancing and quarantine methods to contain the spread of the infection. There are lockdowns all over the world taken as measures to contain its spread. International travel has almost come to a standstill. The situation is really bad causing fear everywhere. Businesses are crumbling. It is not easy to give a lost loved one a good decent send off at a funeral and happy couple have had to postpone their dream weddings. Lifestyles have changed dramatically and drastically. Everyone is asked to wear a mask for protection as it is a highly infectious disease. This is a war against a virus that all of us have come up against. This is the Covid 19 Pandemic which is a universal topic where we hear bad news day by day the world over. Succinctly put, the world today is in a state of gloom and doom a very challenging time. It is a terrible, horrifying, devastating and extremely difficult time and when we will get out of it is wholly uncertain and even whether we will get out of it is yet another question. Those tested positive with

Corona Virus infection, well some have mild symptoms that need to be addressed medically but some others are so serious they are in Intensive Care Unit (ICU) and many thousands round the globe have succumbed to the illness and lost their lives. There is currently no vaccine against Covid 19 A sorry state of affairs.

Legislation are rapidly being enacted and changing every day to keep up with the current situation so that strict measures are being implemented to protect the citizens of affected countries In Singapore we have the Covid 19 (Temporary Measures) Control Order Regulations 2020. One thing is leading to another in this devastation as businesses are collapsing and people are asked to stay home. The slogan of the day from all governments of affected nations around the globe is STAY HOME STAY HOME ADOPT SELF DISTANCING MEASURES AND SELF QUARANTINE. Also, to follow strict rules of hygiene, to wash hands and keep them sanitized and to make sure masks are used when going out to buy essential goods like food and groceries. Jobs are being lost, money hard to come by, so poverty is knocking at the doorstep for a cross section of society who are in any case not very well off. There is economic hardship during this Covid 19 crisis. Therefore, it is becoming hard to feed mouths too for some.

FOREIGN WORKERS IN SINGAPORE

There has been perturbing issues arising on the arena of how foreign construction workers who come from China, Bangladesh, Pakistan and India are being treated and the Covid 19 crisis has been an eye opener to governments to give them additional support. They are an army of a low paid community who come to places like Singapore and the Middle East to earn meager wages to send back home to their families. The cramped dormitories in which the foreign workers reside has proved to be a breeding ground for Covid 19 An explosion of the spread of Corona Virus happened with the foreign workers community in Singapore They are a community of people who have been crucial in the building of Singapore Perhaps there are lessons to learn from this and help is coming from all quarters from the more fortunate showing that the milk of human kindness still flows from the rich, and the mega rich to uplift the living conditions of the foreign workers and to make sure they are counted. It is so important to be humane to all cross sections of society and this is definitely a wake-up call. This has been a blind spot in Singapore. The living conditions of these people are not acceptable and hygiene is not at all in practice. One sees that Mother Nature has been abused through this cross section of people and Singapore is now on a world stage on how it makes amends to the foreign workers. There is a dire need for their conditions to be uplifted and as soon as possible. It appears that Mother Nature is graceful and she has rebelled to bring light to this area.

However trust the Singapore government to take cognizance of their shortcomings and make it better and they will most definitely alleviate the conditions of the foreign workers. After all, the Singapore government has governance based on sound, good and lofty principles but there is no denying that a glaring error has been made. The Singapore Government has recognized it and is swiftly rectifying the situation Now there is testing, isolation and treatment going on and fortunately the foreign workers who are afflicted are young and resilient enough to bounce with back with good health. The Singapore government does run the country with their heart in the right place however this has been a grave omission and Mother Nature has bite back. In life no matter how intelligent one is it is a fallacy to say one knows everything. It is important to apply wisdom and there is a huge difference between wisdom and intellect. Wisdom is the beautiful blend of intellect and spirituality. It is not about chasing money being materialistic earning a huge salary and enjoying life eating Kobe beef in a 7 star hotel and flying private jets or 1st class it is about using money for good causes and uplifting the lives of the less fortunate. That is what makes a truly wholesome character and therein is true success. It is a social responsibility on all of us to care and uplift as far as possible within our capacity, lives of people who are in need. Sadly, there is a large disparity of in the general cross section of society and on the wealth one has. There is an unfair, unequal distribution of wealth the world over therefore, the onus in on the rich to help the poor or other minority groups who are challenged financially or otherwise. This way there will be a better balance and Mother Nature will not be abused as every living being is a creation of Mother Nature deserving of a life of dignity. This foreign domestic issue problem is a reset button as Mother Nature has pushed us to the edge. It is a humbling lesson. Whilst this community of foreign workers built some magnificent buildings in Singapore like Marina Bay Sands and many of us were enjoying dinners at the high-end restaurants with an expensive glass of Champagne, sinfully wasting money in the casino, no one spared a thought for this cross section of society. Many of us were carried away with material success and today the issue of the foreign worker's plight has hit headlines on the conditions they live in. This powerful Corona Virus has taught lessons that we need to learn for life and that is, not to let material success get to our heads but to extend a hand to the underdog. Whilst we are all forced to stay home and work from the home perhaps this is a time to pause, reflect and assimilate wisdom in our lives. Think of the less fortunate, then act on it and lend a helping hand. Not just dash off in the rat race to make and chase money only for personal enjoyment. Is this food for thought? Corona Virus dubbed as an enemy of humanity can also be the biggest teacher if we learn to inculcate supreme values such as having a nobler vision and mission to life. Arrogance based on material success is not proper, correct or acceptable. There has been abuse here on the issue of foreign workers which has to be addressed immediately. Mother Nature is fair, graceful, benevolent and magnanimous and she is teaching us to change our values. And, once that falls into place perhaps the lessons needed to be learnt would have been learnt and we will all view life with a different and more meaningful perceptive. Moving forward, in time, we will see a better tomorrow where foreign workers, their voices of deep suffering and anguish will be heard and they will have a more bearable lifestyle touched by humane understanding and caring. The cry of Mother Nature appears to be at this juncture is to make the necessary changes for this cross section of society and so it will be done. It must be impressed on everyone that they too are human and not to be looked down upon.

There are times one has to be humble and accept the mistakes and make amends and the onus is on all of us to support our government in order to support the foreign workers and not be malicious and caustic in our criticisms. We look forward to a better tomorrow for the foreign workers. When the government has accepted their shortcomings don't put salt on the wound but instead allow the wound to heal so that the nation and the foreign workers can see a healthier tomorrow. We all should stand united in our battle against Covid 19 then we can eventually win.

Plans are under way to improve the living conditions of the foreign workers in fact the BBC commentator said the foreign workers in Singapore are grateful for what the government of Singapore is doing for them. Also, since then, there has been a flow of medical supplies and food supplies to uplift the conditions of the foreign workers in Singapore the government in Singapore has gone all out to tackle this issue with gusto. Aggressive swab testing is going on, on a daily basis to nip the problem in the bud and ensure this community of people are also well cared for and are safe and protected from this deadly disease. Though critics have said otherwise, it can be seen the Singapore government has been relentless in their efforts. For that matter Singapore is doing their best and their utmost during this crisis. The nature of this disease appears to be unscrupulous bringing a lot of suffering to those afflicted and also to those helping the afflicted, be it the government or the medical workers and others involved in the battle against Covid 19. Credit must therefore be given for their selfless efforts to contain further spread of this pandemic and helping those affected...Fortunately a majority of affected foreign workers have only mild symptoms and this can be attributed to early detection with the government's arduous effort in aggressive swab testing.

CIRCUIT BREAKER

As of the date of writing this chapter of this book 27th April 2020 it is to be noted that Singapore went into circuit breaker mode on 7th April

2020. Initially, it was up to 4th May but it has now been extended till 1st of June 2020. This in the context of the current Covid 19 crisis means places of work have shut down island wide except for essential services. Essential services comprise of obtaining food from the food stalls by way of take away banking and mailing items or seeking medical attention. It is mandatory to wear a mask now when you go out with the exception if you are under 2 years of age or you are exercising like running. Beaches that have been frequented by citizens are now closed and so too sports complexes. Private social gatherings as well as public gatherings are strictly prohibited. If you stay together as a family in one household that is fine but not if you are visiting another family member in another household. As of 21st April, less important standalone stalls selling beverages like bubble tea and snacks and confectionaries are also to close down till 1st June 2020. Hair saloons, barber, nail salons excluding health related matters are to close till June 1st 2020. Vacations overseas are now out of the question as most countries abroad are also under lock down. Schools have closed so students have to go into virtual learning.

THE BENEVOLENCE OF SINGAPOREANS

Generous solidarity funds were granted to Singaporeans of $600 each on April 14th 2020 and further solidarity funds granted to businesses to keep them afloat during this difficult time. People are encouraged to work from the home. The hustle and bustle of Singapore's city life has seen a burst in the bubble bring things to a grinding halt. You can only go out to buy groceries and food which you have to take away. Free for All, a charity, founded in 2014, continued to pump in resources delivering food and groceries to elderly and low-income residents amid the circuit breaker. They say more people have requested for food. Community care services such as Meals on Wheels (MOW) remain in service. The MOW program is run by the Agency for Integrated Care (AIC) and delivers on a daily basis 5,300meals. Food from The Heart sends out 7,500 food parcels monthly to the needy. Singaporeans continue to help their fellow citizens

HOW DID COVID 19 START

Covid 19 is believed to have its origins from Wuhan China seafood market. Here wild animals such as marmots, birds, rabbits, bats and snakes, have been illegally sold. Some of them had adopted the undesirable practice of incorporating these species of animal in their diet and so Corona viruses are known to spread from animals to humans As a consequence of this unnatural way of eating the first few people infected with the disease were a group predominantly made up of stallholders from the seafood market. Experts of virologists at the Wuhan Institute for Virology recorded that the new corona viruses', 96 per cent of its constitution genetically is identical to that of a corona virus found in bats

The Wuhan market has since been shut down for inspection and a clean up process on January 1 2020. However, it had proven too late as the damage has been done and it appears that Covid-19 was already starting to spread beyond the market itself. On January 21, according to the WHO Western Pacific office, it was elicited that the disease was also being transmitted between humans. There was evidence that medical staff were infected with the virus. Wuhan, a city state in Eastern China has a population of 11 million. It was on December 31st 2019 that the World Health Organization of China became aware that there was an unfamiliar virus akin to pneumonia that arose in China. In the earlier days, since this disease emanated, Covid 19 was also known as the Wuhan Virus

SYMPTOMS OF COVID 19

COVID-19 affects people in differing ways. Usually infected people will have mild to moderate symptoms.

The following symptoms indicate that you should seek medical attention and get a swab test to see if you are positive

fever.
tiredness.
dry cough.

Shortness of breath
aches and pains.
nasal congestion.
runny nose.
sore throat.
diarrhea.

Normally it takes 5–6 days from the time the person is infected with the virus for symptoms to surface. It can also be up to 14 days when it really shows up.

It is advised that if you have mild symptoms and otherwise feel healthy you should self-isolate. Immediately, see a doctor if you have a fever, a cough, and find it difficult to breathe. The symptoms of COVID-19 infection are akin to regular pneumonia. Typical symptoms include fever, cough and shortness of breath.

PROTECTION AGAINST COVID 19

For the protection of the spread of COVID-19:

Clean your hands frequently. Use soap and water, or alcohol-based hand sanitizers.

Keep a safe distance from anyone who is coughing or sneezing.

Avoid touching your eyes, nose or mouth.

Make sure your nose and mouth are covered with your bent elbow or a tissue when you cough or sneeze.

If you are unwell seek medical attention immediately. If you have, a cough, and difficulty breathing these are symptoms you should not ignore.

Adhere to the laws of your country in regard to safe distancing, lockdown

measures and self quarantine.

WHAT HAPPENS WHEN YOU GET COVID 19?

Older people, and people with pre-existing medical conditions (such as asthma, diabetes, heart disease) are more vulnerable to being severely ill with the virus. In the worse case scenario, they succumb to the illness and die. People with COVID-19 develop mild respiratory symptoms and fever, on an average of 5-6 days after incubation period of infection. Normally people infected with COVID-19 virus have mild disease and recover. However there has been a large death toll in the world as a result of Covid 19.

HOW DOES COVID 19 SPREAD?

The virus that causes COVID-19 is spread through droplets when an infected person coughs, sneezes, or speaks. As the droplets are too heavy to hang in the air they rapidly fall on floors or surfaces. A person can be infected by breathing in the virus. If one is within 1 meter of a person who has COVID-19, or by contacting a contaminated surface and following that they touch their eyes, nose or mouth before washing their hands then one is likely to get infected.

THE SEVERITY OF COVID 19 INFECTIONS – ADDITIONAL MEDICAL INFORMATION

The numbers of COVID-19 infections are on the rise globally. What is alarming is that there seems to be a domino effect and health can spiral down with this infection leading to other complications. There have been an increasing number of reports of neurological symptoms. Reports indicate that over a third of patients are now developing, in addition, neurological symptoms.

In the majority of cases, COVID-19 is a respiratory infection resulting in fever, aches, tiredness, sore throat, cough However recent studies have shown that that COVID-19 can also infect cells outside of the respiratory tract. This can result in range of symptoms from gastrointestinal disease (diarrhea and nausea) to heart damage and blood clotting disorders. Research suggests that neurological symptoms need to be added to this list.

COVID-19 cases have led to neurological symptoms. These studies symptoms have been in some individuals. Numerous reports have described COVID-19 patients suffering from Guillain–Barré syndrome. This is a neurological disorder where the immune system responds to an infection and erroneously attacks nerve cells, with the end result of muscle weakness and eventually paralysis.

Further studies have indicated serious COVID-19 encephalitis (brain inflammation and swelling) and stroke in healthy young individuals with otherwise mild COVID-19 symptoms.

Records from China and France have also shown the existence of neurological disorders in COVID-19 patients. There are records that patients have neurological symptoms.

Disorientation, inattention and movement disorders were also seen in severe cases and found to continue after recovery.

SARS-CoV-2, the corona virus that causes COVID-19, may result in neurological disorders by directly infecting the brain affecting the immune system. These are the studies found in the novel corona virus in the brains people who have died from COVID-19. It appears infection of olfactory neurons in the nose causes the virus to spread from the respiratory tract to the brain.

The human brain has cells in the ACE2 protein on their surface. The endothelial cells are the ACE 2 protein that line blood vessels.

Infection of endothelial cells can pass to the brain from the respiratory tract and when that happens the virus may cause neurological disorders.

On the upside, fortunately, respiratory viruses getting into the brain seldom occurs. One needs a word of caution as so many millions of COVID-19 infections worldwide, run a risk of significant neurological disease, and in serious cases it cannot be ruled out. The neurological manifestations of COVID-19 are a possibility both during severe illness and having long-term effects. It points out the need to protect against and prevent COVID 19 infections Medical experts in China and the US record that the virus that causes Covid-19 can cause the T cells to perish which protect the body from harmful invaders. One doctor said there is growing concerns in the medical fraternity that this spiraling domino effect of the infection could be similar to HIV

SEVERE CASES OF COVID 19

The Covid-19 pandemic is relentless. Now as of writing this book, 27th April 2020, it has reached over 2.7 million cases with over 209,000 deaths. Pharmaceutical companies are doing their very best to find treatments to lessen the gravity of the symptoms of the disease. They are trying to improve on the survival rate of the severely afflicted patients. Several drugs are the subject of deep and extensive research They are trying to reduce acute respiratory distress syndrome (ARDS), a cause of death in Covid-19 patients.

In some Covid-19 patients, the virus triggers the production of inflammatory molecules called cytokines, which results in a "cytokine storm." The lungs fill with water and become intolerant to oxygen, resulting in failure through the intervention of mechanical ventilation resulting in inability to rescue these patients.

Proper treatment for acute respiratory distress syndrome for the severely affected portion of the Covid-19 patients is the answer to decreasing the mortality of the disease. Research shows one in six Covid-19 patients suffer from difficulty in breathing, and 40% of those who have difficulty in breathing develop ARDS. There is only a 20% -50% survival rate of ARDS patients, treated with mechanical ventilation. Currently extensive research is ongoing to find the proper medical treatment to Covid 19

WHO (World Health Organization) ON SMOKING AND COVID 19?

Some French Scientist have postulated a theory that smoking can combat the spread of Covid 19. However, WHO refutes this theory and does not endorse their views it is to be noted.

COUNTRIES WITH NO COVID19 INFECTIONS

According to the record kept by the Johns Hopkins University corona virus resource center out of 200 or so countries and territories in the world, 181 have reported at least one case COVID-19. The pandemic, has spread across the world rapidly and alarmingly. Covid 19 is almost everywhere.

The Solomon Islands, Vanuatu, Samoa, Kiribati, Micronesia, Tonga, the Marshall Islands Palau, Tuvalu, and Nauru appear to be spared of COVID-19. These countries have restricted travel and have implemented steps to prevent and protect against the arrival or spread of the virus.

COUNTRIES CURRENTLY EASING ON LOCKDOWN

Denmark, Germany, Switzerland and Austria are among the European countries are putting an ease to their lockdown. Schools and shops are reopening – but leaders are aware that this requires a proper balancing act.

The curves have flattened and infection rates of the COVID-19 are making a decline in their cases. Some European countries are easing their societies back towards normalcy of daily life. Also, some good news the numbers of new infections in Italy, France and Spain continue to decrease. These countries are in the process of easing their lockdowns. Shops and factories will be first to resume work.

Now, three of the world's hardest-hit nations, are preparing to lift the restrictions in their attempts to stop the spread of COVID-19.

US being the forerunner, the countries next on the list of -highest numbers of confirmed cases - Spain, Italy and France - have made announcements that they plan for a cautious gradual exit of their lockdowns. Also, amongst these countries to ease the lockdown are Norway, Iran, Czech Republic, Austria, China, Sweden and New Zealand. Singapore is also planning to ease off on its circuit breaker but the government has warned that it does not mean we should let our guard down and be complacent as the battle is not yet over.

Let's hope for victory and slowly and surely the world over, to come out of this dark, sinister and sordid tunnel. May the resplendent rays of the glorious sun shine through. Let there be a breaking of a new dawn after this terrible storm for humanity at large

MORE GOOD NEWS AWAITS YOU IN THE NEXT AND FINAL CHAPTER

There is some positive information in the next chapter on the preventive and protective methods you can use to combat Covid 19 and that too not just Covid 19 but all viruses. GoodAire Pte Ltd of which the author of this book Richard Yeck, is the inventor, brings you a host of products which have been manufactured through years of scientific research to keep Covid 19 away. The fight against the epidemic of SARS subscribed to the products of Good Aire Pte Ltd and the company has emerged with great success and has a proven track record. Through arduous research refining and evolving their hard ware and software they now embark to take on the monumental task of protecting against the spread of COVID 19 and can deliver the goods.

It is reiterated that it is not a cure but a preventive and protective measure to contain the spread of Covid 19 spread. It is not medical science but delves in the area of environmental science. The chapter unlocks secrets of the inventor's research on how you can sanitize your hands, purify and disinfect the air your breathe and keep your surrounding clear and clean and prevent the spread of Covid 19. Richard Yeck subscribes to the theory that you need a clean environment so that viruses do not breed. We hope to get out of this phase in time and make Covid 19 history one day.

CHAPTER 3

UNIQUE METHODS FROM GOODAIRE SANZ TO PROTECT AGAINT BACTERIA, GERMSAND COMBAT COVID 19 VIRUS

THE HISTORY OF GOODAIRE SANZ AND RICHARD YECK'S IINVENTIONS

GoodAire Pte Ltd brings to you a breath of fresh air and a ray of hope in this battle against Covid 19 virus. No, it is not a vaccine that promises a cure neither is it a medical science discovery. It is related to environmental science and whilst it does not promise or propagate a cure it puts forward unique measures to protect and prevent against the spread of the virus. It is really pertinent and relevant in today's condition of the bleak and gloomy world.

Richard Yeck is an Inventor and the Founder of GoodAire Pte Ltd

The company was born out of an inspiration to uplift the suffering conditions of humanity when epidemics and pandemics strike. Life of GoodAire Pte Ltd began in 2003 when he had a brainwave when he once saw an airline stewardess spraying the cabin with an air freshener.

Inspired, he thought why not manufacture a device that would suck up pollutants and revitalise the air?

And thus, GoodAire air revitaliser, was born and launched that year the percentage of clean air is increased it is allergy-free and conducive for asthmatics and people with sinus issues. Since then, Good Aire Pte Ltd has made great inroads in groundbreaking and revolutionary products that act as deterrents to the spread of various germs, bacteria and viruses that cause illnesses to mankind. Richard Yeck is the brains behind GoodAire Sanz and he is a one man show that researches, develops and evolves his products to create a better environment making it clean from the spread of viruses, bacteria and germs. He does however exchange views with eminent virus and environmental scientist. The main thrust and underlying principles in the production of these products is to ensure a clean free from pollution and contaminants environment.

Today, Good Aire Pte Ltd produces user friendly air humidifiers, air purifiers, sanitizers, and masks to contain the spread of Covid 19 virus. The company has over the years developed an impeccable reputation and a proven track record. Their products to clean up the environment and keep it safe from spread of Covid 19 virus, other germs, other viruses and bacteria are genuine and worthy of serious consideration. With his deep research and extensive studies Richard Yeck says referring to Covid 19.

Richard Yeck invented The First Air Purifier to Knock Out Mosquitoes

Did you ever think that you can clean and humidify the air, get rid of pesky mosquitoes, diffuse fragrant aromas, and provide ambient lighting to your room with just one product? Also you can use a palm-sized atomizer to repel mosquitoes while you are out camping, Richard Yeck is a pioneer of multi functional air purifying products

With GoodAire's revolutionary **5-in-1 Air Revitalizer H1 and Atomizer P1**, you now can achieve this

"The best part about our products is that they are all natural. We draw on nature's best resources — water and essential oils — to resolve the growing threats

of mosquito and mosquito-related diseases as well as polluted air." – Richard Yeck, Founder of GoodAire

GoodAire Air Revitalizer H1 During SARS Period in 2003

I developed the first generation GoodAire Air Revitalizer, and I was propelled by the overwhelming market response to the product. It was a phenomenal success when it was launched during the SARs period in 2003. By cleansing and disinfecting the air, this product effectively removed germs and other impurities in the environment.

After my initial success with the first generation of the Air Revitalizer, I encountered various set backs in the years after.

I plodded on and my spirit kept me going though I felt like giving up a times. However, it was during this time that. I acquired a deeper insight of the science of using water as a purification system.

Dengue and Zika

'I' was keen on solving the problem of mosquitoes, especially with cases of Dengue and Zika on the rise in Singapore and the region. I therefore spent the next ten years researching the use of essential oils against mosquitoes, while at the same time fine-tuning the water filtering technology.

This resulted in a multi-functional, intelligent air cleansing and mosquito repelling system.

My mission, succinctly, is to provide clean air and a safe home environment for families to enjoy and thrive – especially those with elderly parents or young children in their homes.

I was well aware that we live in a high-density urban environment where air pollution is constantly affecting our lives.

With the rise of allergies in children (eczema, asthma, you name it) and their negative reactions toward dust-mites, pet dander (microscopic specks of skin shed by pet birds and animals), and pollen from flowering plants, it is imperative that we raise our standards of clean air for everyone, and make it easily attainable for families who need it most'.

Air Revitalizer H1 and Atomizer P1 gets rid of mosquitoes

The GoodAire Air Revitalizer H1 combines a water-based filtration system with nano vent technology. The nano vent technology eliminates liquid mess and slowly diffuses essential oil blends into the air via nano-porous beads.

Like the Air Revitalizer H1, the GoodAire Atomizer P1 makes use of nano vent technology to slowly diffuse essential oil into the water solution via nano-porous beads. The only difference is that it works by spraying fine mists of natural oil infused water into the air, helping to drive away mosquitoes.

Both products allow the air to stay cleaner and fresher for hours. The scent from our Moz Defence nano vent cartridge series lingers in the air, and renders mosquitoes immobilized. Our lab tests show that 100% of the mosquitoes are knocked down within 2-5 minutes.

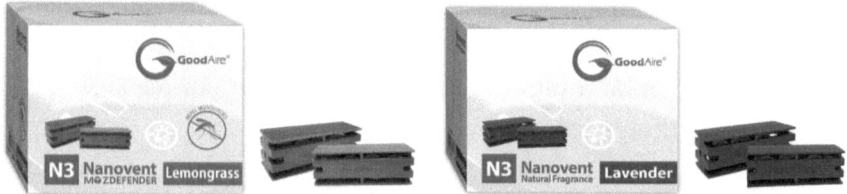

The most unique aspect of the GoodAire Air Revitalizer H1

That would be the unique air and water-flow system that we designed and patented. The technology behind it is premised on the simple idea of using water and a rotating impeller to create a high-speed water curtain to "scrub" and cleanse the air of impurities.

Another distinctive aspect of the product is the use of nanovent technology to enable a slow diffusion process of essential oils into the clean air. The result is an environment that stays cleaner and fresher (and even mosquito-free) for longer periods of time. It is all natural and easy to use; just swap in a new cartridge when the old one is spent.

Where the Air Revitalizer H1 and the Atomizer P1 can be used

The GoodAire Air Revitalizer H1 can be used in any room with access to an electrical point. They include the living rooms and bedrooms of homes, hospital wards, clinics, offices, factories, classrooms and even dormitories and hostel rooms.

Easily rechargeable using USB power source, the GoodAire Atomizer P1 is suitable for outdoor uses. You can bring it along for camping in tents, in the army barracks, in dormitories, or when you are outdoors.

Future plans in terms of product design

We are in the process of developing a full range of Air Revitalizer products, including a mist fan, air cooler, and humidifier. All of these can be fitted with the Moz Defender nanovent series, for mosquito-repelling capability. We plan to add new natural fragrances to expand the existing range, and we are also working to create new commercial fragrances for the office sector and entertainment outlets.

"My mission is quite simply to provide clean air and a safe home environment for families to enjoy and thrive — especially those with elderly parents or young children in their homes" — Richard Yeck, Founder of GoodAire

"The best part about our products is that they are all natural. We draw on nature's best resources — water and essential oils — to resolve the growing threats of mosquito and mosquito-related diseases as well as polluted air." — Richard Yeck, Founder of GoodAire

The result of this research is a multi-functional, intelligent air cleansing and mosquito repelling system.

"We Draw on Nature's Best Kept Secrets to Care for Your Health"

Inspired by Mother Nature, GoodAire uses a water-based filtration system to purify the air, just like how rain washes the earth's atmosphere. Every raindrop serves to rid the atmosphere of micro-pollutants and replenish the ground and soil with moisture.

Get ready for good clean air with GoodAire's range of air revitalizing and purifying products. GoodAire ensures that all its products are environmentally-friendly and non-ozone producing.

Staying outdoor in the evening has never felt safe for anyone because of mosquitoes, but it is over now. GoodAire mosquito repellent is filled with 100% natural essential oils that repel and knock down mosquitoes in 2 – 5 minutes. It has no chemical and it is safe for both the young and elderly.

The P1 which is the portable pocket-sized atomizer is your on-the-go defense against mosquitoes and airborne bacteria. It creates a mosquito-free zone within minutes as water mixed with essential oils from our patented nanovent cartridges is released as a fine and powerful mist into the air. These droplets repel and knock down mosquitoes in the vicinity, forming an invisible shield around you and your family. Each set comes with 2 Moz Defender water cartridges. Each water cartridge allows for 20 refills of water, and each refill lasts about 4-5 hours. Now you can enjoy the great outdoors with complete peace of mind. It is rechargeable with micro USB and is suitable for camping, hiking, travelling, cars, family time outside. It can used in homes, schools, hospitals and everywhere you go.

The GoodAire Air Revitalizer H1 combines a water-based filtration system with nanovent technology. The nanovent technology eliminates liquid mess and slowly diffuses essential oil blends into the air via nano-porous beads.

Like the Air Revitalizer H1, the GoodAire Atomizer P1 makes use of nanovent technology to slowly diffuse essential oils into the water solution via nano-porous beads. The only difference is that it works by spraying fine mists of natural oil infused water into the air, helping to drive away mosquitoes.

Both products allow the air to stay cleaner and fresher for hours. The fragrance from our MozDefence Nanovent cartridge series lingers in the air, and renders mosquitoes immobilized. Our lab tests show that 100% of the mosquitoes are knocked down within 2-5 minutes.

The best part about our products is that they are all natural. We draw on nature's best resources – water and essential oils to resolve the growing threats of mosquito and mosquito-related diseases as well as polluted air

WHY GOODAIRE MOSQUITO REPELLENTS IN AFRICA?

Malaria is caused by a one-celled parasite called Plasmodium. Female Anopheles. Mosquitoes pick up the parasite from infected people when they bite to obtain blood needed to nurture their eggs. Inside the mosquito the parasites reproduce and develop. When the mosquito bites again, the parasites contained in the salivary gland are injected and passed through the blood of the person being bitten. Malaria parasites multiply rapidly in the liver and then in red blood cells of the infected person. One to two weeks after a person is infected the first symptoms of malaria appear: usually fever, headache, chills and vomiting. If not treated promptly with effective medicines, malaria can kill by infecting and destroying red blood cells and by clogging the capillaries that carry blood to the brain or other vital organs.

There are four types of human malaria: Plasmodium P. vivax, P. malariae, P. ovale and P. falciparum. P. vivax and P. falciparum are the most common forms. Falciparum malaria—the deadliest type—is most common in sub-Saharan Africa, where it causes more than 400 000 deaths a year.

In recent years, some human cases of malaria have also occurred with Plasmodium knowlesi – a specie that causes malaria among monkeys and occurs in certain forested areas of South-East Asia.

About 90% of all malaria deaths in the world today occur in Africa south of the Sahara. This is because the majority of infections in Africa are caused by Plasmodium falciparum, the most dangerous of the four human malaria parasites. It is also because the most effective malaria vector – the mosquito Anopheles gambiae – is the most widespread in Africa and the most difficult to control. An estimated one million people in Africa die from malaria each year and most of these are children under the age of 5. The WHO collaborates with 3 centers world wide for testing of mosquito repellants and they are in Florida America New Delhi India and Penang Malaysia. Richard Yeck through Good Aire Sanz and his products has over the last 10 years been in consultation with these centers to endorse his views and products and they have all been well received. He strongly recommends that Singapore also set up such a centre so that those coming up with products that are not authentic can be taken off the list. Some of them use synthetic fragrances to enhance their products and to make it attractive to the consumer market but Richard Yeck is of the view that this can prove more harmful than useful. It is with pride that Richard Yeck says the fruits of his toil saw glory and that Good Aire Revitaliser earned the Singapore Mosquito Repellent Parent Choice Award in 2018.

RICHARD YECK GOODAIRE SANZ SCIENTIFIC WISDOM IN BATTLING COVID 19

Richard Yeck has through his years of work at GoodAire Pte Ltd emerged as formidable self-made environmental scientist. He has made it to the newspapers on numerous occasions with his impressive track record for bringing out environmental solutions, gadgets and items to combat and prevent several other diseases caused by bacteria and viruses. Though a one man show, he does consult other eminent scientists the world over and his views have been well received, highly respected and endorsed by reputable laboratories. We now leave the platform of his past success and travel into the arena of today's battle against the spread of Covid 19 viruses. We will look in depth at his ingenious proposition and what he postulates are the best theoretical and practical methods in environmental science to contain the spread of Corona Virus. He advocates the use of disinfectants through air humidifiers air purifiers, sanitizers and the mandatory use of masks to stop the spread of the Covid Virus. We will also look at the multitude of his goods which he has developed and evolved through his extensive studies and research. It is interesting to note that he states, "I saw this coming I knew the world was coming in for a pandemic but I was only three quarters prepared when it arrived and I was shocked that it arrived sooner than expected." "Still I battle on to find practical solutions as it is my responsibility to do so. I am propelled by my deep desire and passion to help humanity and not for monetary gains. I am completely committed and dedicated in this battle and my sole mission is to find a solution that will stand to be in good stead along with the research from medical science. My research, contributions and discoveries in environmental science will only supplement the current research that is going on to find a proper vaccine and until that happens I believe Covid 19 is here to stay. My contributions are to curtail the spread and not offer a cure to the disease as that is for the medical scientist to do."

"This is a time when one can't save on one's money one needs to invest in material that will curtail the spread of the Covid 19 virus in order to be safe and protected. "Prevention is better than cure. "Good health is the greatest of wealth. These materials from Good Aire Sanz are genuine and authenticated by reputable laboratories the world over like Australia and China to name some."

SOME CARDINAL RULES TO FOLLOW

Good indoor air quality during the COVID-19 pandemic is a must

Richard Yeck wishes to orchestrate to the world about the importance of maintaining indoor air quality in your home or business during the

COVID-19 pandemic. He says supreme indoor air quality is a gateway to contain the spread of Covid 19 virus. For this Good Aire Pte Ltd has launched Good Aire Sanz, some specific air purifying systems that is worth considering especially now that we are all indoors most of the time due to lockdown. Many of these items act as a disinfectant to you and your home or office.

He points to The Centers for Disease Control and Prevention or CDC r which attributed an outbreak in January to the air conditioning system inside of a restaurant in Guangzhou, China. The WHO has dubbed that when a building is affected adversely due to poor indoor air quality it is called the Sick Building Syndrome. This leads to many other harmful diseases and Covid 19 virus spread is indeed one of them.

He states "This should not come as a surprise as Air Conditioning systems are the perfect breeding ground for viruses such as COVID-19.

He expands "the spread of Covid 19 Virus is exacerbated with predominantly three things.:. That is food, such as the microscopic skin particles we shed every day which float in the air and permeate your A/C system; then moisture, generated through the air conditioning system and the absence of UV light, created by the sun. A combination of all these factors creates a conducive breeding ground for Covid 19 virus."

He says to help preserve the air quality in their homes and businesses, one should keep their air filters air purifiers or air humidifiers clean and change them frequently.

"Your filter operates like face mask for your air conditioning system; It is imperative to keep it clean and change it often. Also get a UV light installed in your air handler and that will it helps control the organic growth in the air handler and keeps the coil clean. The most important thing is to install a whole-home air purification system. I qualify myself in saying that though they have not been tested specifically for COVID-19, they have in the past been tested and [shown to be] 99.9% effective against [H5N1 or] the 'bird flu' and [H1N1 or] the 'swine flu'. It is to be noted that their DNA and RNA viruses are likened to COVID-19 virus"

*Air conditioning had spread the corona virus to 9 people sitting near an infected person in a restaurant. This has huge implications for the service industry as reported on

April 21, 2020

Three healthy families were afflicted by COVID-19 when they dined at neighbouring tables in a windowless restaurant in Guangzhou, China, in January.

Researchers are of the view that the restaurant's _*air conditioner blew the viral droplets of one person who was asymptomatic farther than they might have normally gone*_. Nine other people who were there in the vicinity later got afflicted.

The researchers in the journal Emerging Infectious Diseases described

"It's a frightening prospect for people who are trying to keep a healthy distance from others.

However, in a potentially hopeful finding for the locked-down restaurant industry, none of the 73 other diners and eight employees in the restaurant at the time got sick".

"To prevent the spread of the virus in restaurants, we recommend _ *increasing the distance between tables and improving ventilation*_," they wrote.

According to the Air Conditioning Contractors of America or ACCA, the use ultraviolet lights will not completely rid your home of mold or viruses but results shown when use they have gone a long way and been effective when used correctly.

WHY WEARING A MASK IS MANDATORY IN THE FIGHT AGAINST COVID 19

The Centers for Disease Control and Prevention (CDC) says.

"We now know from recent studies that a significant portion of individuals with Corona virus lack symptoms ("asymptomatic") and that even those who eventually develop symptoms ("pre-symptomatic") can transmit the virus to others before showing symptoms," according to the advisory published by the CDC. "There is medical evidence that the virus can spread between people in close proximity. This includes when people speak, cough, or sneeze — even if people do not exhibit symptoms.

On this premise CDC recommends wearing cloth face coverings in public settings. There are situations when social distancing measures are difficult to maintain (e.g., grocery stores and pharmacies)

The CDC supported its new position by citing several studies about the asymptomatic spread of the disease, the first of which was published on March 5 in the New England Journal of Medicine. New evidence indicate that infected people are likely to spread the virus to others for two to three days before becoming ill, says Associate Professor Hsu Li Yang from Saw Swee Hock School of Public Health in the National University of Singapore. With these findings now in Singapore wearing a mask when you are up and about is mandatory. Incidentally, it is to be noted that Good Aire Sanz is bringing out a mask made of cloth and disinfected with DST+(Nano AG TIO2+) durable for 100 wash.

THE IMPORTANCE OF HAND HYGIENE

Records indicate that thousands of people die every day around the world from infections when receiving health care. • Hands are the main conduit for germ transmission. • Therefore, the most important measure to avoid the transmission of harmful germs and be protected against health care-associated infections. Is through hand hygiene

You should clean your hands by rubbing them with an alcohol-based sanitizer If hands are not visibly dirty it is more effective, by your hands than washing with soap and water. • You must wash your hands with soap and water when hands are visibly dirty. • If there is exposure to potential spore-forming pathogens hand washing with soap and water is the better option.

GOODAIRE SANZ PRESENTS HOLISTIC ENVIROMENTAL SUPPLEMENTS PROTECTING AGAINST SPREAD OF COVID 19 VIRUS

As an established company with a proven track record of killing viruses and bacteria it has now created a hardware and soft ware air purifying system and a complete sanitizing system that can kill the virus in a record breaking 9 seconds(endorsed by Australian Laboratory Services) You can leave these air purifiers /humidifier in your homes (buildings) and be rest assured of adequate protection. It is a simple method of stationing the purifier that has a tablet dissolving in it and the air gets refreshed with cleaner, healthier virus and bacteria free air in the whole surrounding area of your home or building. It is in summary, a total air sanitizing system that works. It uses Chlorine Dioxide (CIO2) a safe and effective disinfectant, DST+(Nano AG TIO2+), and optionally Covalent Ag+-03. To elaborate a little, Chlorine Dioxide is an extremely potent disinfectant that can aggressively kill bacteria, viruses and parasites.

The proven track record of GoodAire Pte Ltd worldwide is that CIO2 complies with all safety concerns of World Health Organization, United States Environmental Protection Agency, Food and Drug Administration and United States Department of Agriculture. Test Reports consists of Bacterial Activity by SGS China, TUV SUD PSB Singapore, ALS Technician (S) Pte Ltd Singapore. Virucidal Activity tested and endorsed by UNIMAS Malaysia and Indoor Air Quality Performance by Axiom Laboratory.

For a total solution to kill the virus and bacteria Mr. Richard Yeck summarizes the following practice

1. Put a disinfected Floor mat as the shoe is the culprit. When it rubs on the floor mat it is disinfected
2. Disinfecting Tent 18 ft (6m)
3. Spray CIO2, DST on entire building
4. Mask is a must
5. Have a big sanitizing unit
6. Uniform groups should have their uniforms washed and treated with DST+ which last a minimum 3 months for per 100 wash
7. Have a vehicle sanitizing unit
8. Use small sanitizers for homes and offices

"I hope I have imparted crystal clear knowledge to you on how Good Air Sanz uses Chlorine Dioxide (CIO2) a safe and effective disinfectant, DST+(Nano AG TIO2+), and optionally Covalent Ag+-03 to disinfect and sanitize every facet of your lifestyle especially now, that you are indoors most of the time. As a picture paints a thousand words, I am including my power point slides to illustrate how it works and it does work to contain the spread of Covid 19virus. Our products are tested by highly reputable laboratories. I hope you will assimilate the contents of this book and act wisely as this war against Covid 19 virus is a deadly war and we need to be vigilant and diligent in our way of life. We need to adapt to the current situation and take cognizance of its seriousness. It is imperative that you act to protect you, your family and your employees and it includes all cross section of society. I would like to impress on all of you that to protect yourselves the onus lies with each one of us.

Our Air Humidifier is a well-designed gadget that serves the purpose fully and the method to use it is simple and very user friendly. The pictures are in the last chapter of this book as it will then certainly impact on you in a big way on the extensive research that is done to protect your health. We work on the motto that "Prevention is better than cure" so protect yourselves and combat Covid 19 through the plethora of wholesome gadgets and effective methods that GoodAire

Sanz has to offer. Rather than battle Covid 19 in the hospital bed we urge you to battle Covid 19 through disinfecting and sanitizing your home your buildings your clothes and other things that need sanitizing and disinfecting through Good Aire Sanz. Better safe than sorry.

It is my humble suggestion that as in the case of the foreign dormitory situation, where the virus has spread to the point of being uncontrollable that a total disinfecting and sanitizing system be used to kill the virus and stop it from breeding any further. Good Aire Sanz is one such product that is highly potent enough to kill the virus in 9 seconds as tested by a reputable laboratory. Perhaps investing in Good Aire Sanz is the gateway to better environmental health and can contain the spread of Covid 19 virus. It has a real and dynamic answer to contain any further breeding of this contagious infection." Richard Yeck

As of the date of publication of this book 24th May 2020 the figures for Corona Virus worldwide stand as stated below

Confirmed	Recovered	Deaths
5.31M	**2.11M**	**342K**
+110K		+5,676

ANNEXTURE

AN INTERESTING READ FROM EMINENT SCIENTISTS IN SINGAPORE

Possible transmission mechanisms of SARS-Cov-2
Dr Patrick Fernandez FRACI
Pacific-Tec Scientific P/L

On 11 March 2020, the World Health Organization (WHO) declared the coronavirus disease 2019 (COVID-19) a worldwide pandemic. SARS-CoV-2, the virus responsible for this, generally spreads by human-to-human transmission via droplets or direct person to person contact. Infections can also spread by touching surfaces and objects that have been contaminated with virus-containing droplets released from an infected person. Additionally, since SARS-CoV-2 (as well as other coronaviruses) had been found in fecal samples and anal swabs of some patients, and of late even in the semen of men, the possibility of fecal-oral (including waterborne) transmission needs further understanding.

This short review whilst not exhaustive provides an insight into possible mechanisms of transmission via air, fomites and water. We examine the factors that make this possible with references to the literature, drawing upon studies in published reviews (and from which other citations are made). Let us start with a basic understanding of the external structure and form of the SARS-CoV-2 virus and how this facilitates air, fomite or water borne transmission.

External structure and form of SARS-CoV-2 virus

SARS-CoV-2 comes from the family of corona viruses. Coronaviruses (CoVs) are enveloped viruses with the RNA genome. These viruses enclose their genomes inside a lipid bilayer which is filled with various proteins that facilitate virus entry into target human cells.

SARS-CoV-2 is spherical, and about 120 nm in diameter. It is generally expelled together with mucous. However, as the envelope is fragile, anything which causes its breakage exposing its internal components can cause it to degrade.

Air transmission

WHO has recommended hand washing with soap and water, whilst maintaining social distancing as the main measures to lessen the probability of getting infected or spreading Covid-19. Infection however is still possible by inhalation of small droplets released by an infected person. Studies have shown that air borne droplets can travel meters or tens of meters in the air with their viral content. We examine here this transport mechanism and the evidence how this is a significant route of infection.

Morawska and Cao (2020), have conducted a comprehensive review of this air borne route in some detail. As soon as an infected person expels droplets of viral laden mucous, notably through sneezing, coughing or breathing, the liquid within can quickly start to evaporate. Subsequently, some droplets may become so small that they are affected more by air currents than falling to the ground. These small droplets with their viral contents may then travel in the air tens of meters from where an infected individual is located.

Morawska et al (2009) also studied the size distribution of droplets expelled from the human respiratory tract during expiratory activities e.g. when talking, droplets were just a few microns in size. Li et al (2005) cited a study by Duguid (1945) and reported that sneezing and coughing could generate a

million or so droplets up to 100 μm in diameter in conjunction with several thousand larger particles. They studied the role of air distribution in SARS transmission during the largest nosocomial outbreak in Hong Kong in 2003. Humid droplets, upon release start to evaporate changing their mass and size. Droplet sizes could shrink to as small 0.5–12 μm to be airborne.

Likewise, large particles settling because of gravity could be resuspended as they evaporated and became smaller. This rate of evaporation was largely dependent on the ambient humidity. In indoor air-conditioned environments controlled with 50-60% relative humidity, sizes of droplets with diameters of less than 100 μm can quickly shrunk once released into the air.

Air velocity, air temperature and relative humidity can directly affect such situations, and these are applicable both in indoor or outdoor settings. We should endeavour to minimize air borne transmission especially in indoor environments. Increasing the ventilation rate, for example by natural means, the avoidance of recirculating air and staying away from another person's direct air flow, whilst minimizing the number of people in an enclosed space are all important considerations. Where possible, the maximization of natural ventilation in purpose-built buildings or modifications to facilitate natural ventilation to ensure high ventilation rates should be encouraged.

Transmission via fomites

Fomite transmission often involves a secondary route (via non-living objects) of exposure through oral or direct contact for viruses to enter the host.

These include non-living surfaces, such as counter tops or doorknobs, as well as objects, like clothing or house hold utensils. Dust particles containing the virus can circulate in the air after droplets of infected mucous are sneezed or coughed into the air are also examples of fomites. Another common example of a fomite requiring some vigilance, could be a park water fountain from which many people drink. Viral containing mucous deposited by one person can potentially be transmitted to subsequent users.

Boone and Gerba (2007) did an interesting review and cited various studies to assess the significance of fomites in the transmission of viral respiratory disease. Fomites consist of both porous (cloth, paper) and nonporous surfaces or objects (metal, hard plastics, tile) and once virus contaminated can become transmission vehicles. During the course of an infection, viruses can be released in large numbers through various body secretions e.g. blood, feces, urine, saliva, and nasal fluid. Possible transmission of infection can occur through contact with these secretions, through breathing in aerosolized virus expelled via talking, sneezing, coughing, or even contact with airborne virus that settles after disturbance of a contaminated fomite (i.e., shaking a contaminated bed sheet or blanket).

Once contamination occurs, the infectious virus may readily transfer between humans and objects or between two separate fomites (if brought together), before infecting someone.

During an outbreak of infectious disease, it is not uncommon to see rapid spread in an indoor setting. Schools, day care facilities, nursing homes, business offices, and hospitals, are prime targets.

The potential for a viral spread via contaminated fomites depends on its ability to maintain infectivity. Once contact is established with a potential host, viral entry can occur through the mouth, nose, and eyes. However, whether the host succumbs to the disease is dependent on previous contact with the virus and the strength of the host current immune system.

van Doremalen et al (2020) reported viral decay for SARS-CoV-2 on fomites, was faster in copper and cardboard compared to that on plastic and stainless steel (detected up to 72 hours) after application. On copper, no viable presence measured after 4 hours whilst on cardboard none was measured after 24 hours.

The length of time a virus remains active can depend on notably temperature, humidity and the environmental surrounding. In general, UV exposure and pH have minimal effects on viral survival in indoor environments. An interesting observation was viral survival was influenced by the number of microbes present on a surface, which can serve to protect viruses from desiccation and disinfection. Typically, viral presence on fomites may decrease with surface cleanliness. However, it was noticed that some cleaning products or disinfectants could be ineffective against viruses and can result in viral spread or cross-contamination of surfaces.

Boone and Gerba (2007) cited several disease outbreaks where fomites were the culprit as potential transmission vehicles. During an outbreak in a Honolulu nursing home, it was determined that hands of staff or fomites (e.g., towels, medical cart items, etc.) spread the influenza virus. Studies in day care centers have detected rotavirus on various surfaces, including toys, phones, toilet handles, sinks, and water fountains. A hospital in Taiwan in 2003 detected coronavirus on hospital phones, doorknobs, computer mouses, and toilet handles during an outbreak of severe acute respiratory syndrome (SARS).

Water borne transmission

La Rosa et al (2020) reported of the detection of SARS-CoV-2 in sewage in Europe, USA and Australia. The detection of the virus in sewage, albeit when there is little evidence of this, indicates that sewage monitoring could be a good barometer to gauge the circulation of the virus in a community.

Liu and Naddeo (2020) reported that viruses can be transported in microscopic water droplets, or aerosols, entering the air through evaporation or sprays and then falling into various water sources. It is apparent however, whether this pathway represents a threat will depend on the virus ability to persist and survive. They reported than it is known that coronaviruses, including the SARS-CoV-2 virus can remain infectious for days or even longer in sewage and drinking water.

If we examine past studies carried out, we can find some evidence of this. During the 2003 SARS outbreak in Hong Kong, a sewage leak caused a cluster of cases through aerosolization. Though no known cases of COVID-19 have been caused by sewage leaks, the SARS-Cov-2 virus is closely related to the one that causes SARS, and infection via this route could be possible.

It is thought that this virus can colonize biofilms (but the extent to which they can happen has not yet been studied) that line drinking water systems, making showerheads a possible source of aerosolized transmission. Legionnaire's disease caused by a bacterial infection, is thought to be transmitted via this pathway. Biofilms are thin, slimy bacterial growths that often line the pipes of many aging drinking water systems.

Most countries have stringent water treatment routines and these are thought to kill or remove coronaviruses effectively in both drinking and wastewater. Disinfection processes involving oxidation with hypochlorous acid or peracetic acid, and ultraviolet irradiation, as well as chlorine, are thought to kill coronaviruses. The breakage of the viral envelope will lead to the loss of key functional receptors required for cellular infection, and its subsequent demise. Additionally, as wastewater treatment plants use membrane bioreactors, beneficial microorganisms and filter suspended solids, viruses harbouring in sewage sludge, can be eliminated.

Liu and Naddeo (2020) also suggest upgrading existing water and wastewater treatment facilities in hot areas having viral outbreaks, with noticeably high viral loads such at hospitals, community clinics, and nursing homes. In such instances, additional precautions could be to disinfect outflows using light-emitting, ultraviolet systems before it enters the public water systems.

La Rosa et al (2020) cited the study of Wang et al (2005) who studied the persistence of SARS-CoV in hospital wastewater, domestic sewage, and dechlorinated tap water. They detected the viral presence in tap water for 2 days at 20 °C and up to 14 days at 4 °C.

In general, in the various types of water tested, the quantity of infectious virus declined more rapidly at 25 °C than at 4 °C, confirming that temperature is an important factor affecting viral survival and persistence in water.

Another interesting finding of the study was that coronavirus inactivation was faster in filtered tap water than unfiltered tap water, suggesting that suspended solids in water can provide protection for viruses adsorbed to these particles.

Conclusions

Respiratory viruses like SARS-Cov-2 typically cause sneezing and coughing, potentially expelling large amounts of infectious virions to travel to distances greater than 3 m and contaminate surrounding fomites. A combination of air and fomite transmission is perhaps one area which needs careful monitoring.

Coronaviruses show high sensitivity to disinfectants in water. Current data tends to suggest that public drinking-water supplies are safe for consumption and standard treatment protocols, such as filtration and disinfection are effective against coronaviruses.

References

Robert Stass, Weng M. Ng, Young Chan Kim, Juha T. Huiskonen
Structures of enveloped virions determined by cryogenic electron microscopy and tomography
Advances in Virus Research, Volume 105, 2019, Pages 35-71

M. Alejandra Tortorici, David Veesler
Chapter Four - Structural insights into coronavirus entry
Advances in Virus Research, Volume 105, 2019, Pages 93-116

Lidia Morawska, Junji Cao
Airborne transmission of SARS-CoV-2: The world should face the reality
Environment International, 139 (2020)

L. Morawska, G.R. Johnson, Z.D. Ristovski, M. Hargreaves, K. Mengersen, S. Corbett, C.Y.H. Chao, Y. Li, D. Katoshevski.

Size distribution and sites of origin of droplets expelled from the human respiratory tract during expiratory activities

Journal of Aerosol Science, Volume 40, Issue 3, March 2009, Pages 256-269

Y. Li, X. Huang, I. T. S. Yu, T. W. Wong, H. Qian
Role of air distribution in SARS transmission during the largest nosocomial outbreak in Hong Kong
Indoor Air 2005, Volume 15, Issue 2

Stephanie A. Boone* and Charles P. Gerba
Significance of Fomites in the Spread of Respiratory and Enteric Viral Disease
Applied and Environmental Microbiology. 2007 Mar; 73(6): 1687–1696.

Neeltje van Doremalen et al
Aerosol and Surface Stability of SARS-CoV-2 as Compared with SARS-CoV-1
New England Journal of Medicine 2020; 382:1564-1567

Duguid, J.F. (1945)
The numbers and the sites of origin of the droplets expelled during expiratory activities, Edinburg Med. J., 52, 385– 401.

Giuseppina La Rosa, Lucia Bonadonna, Luca Lucentini, Sebastien Kenmoe, Elisabetta Suffredini

Coronavirus in water environments: Occurrence, persistence and concentration methods - A scoping review.

Water Research 179 (2020), 115899.

Xin-Wei Wang, Jin-Song Li, Min Jin, Bei Zhen, Qing-Xin Kong, Nong Song, Wen-Jun Xiao, Jing Yin, Wei Wei, Gui-Jie Wang, Bing-yin Si, Bao-Zhong Guo, Chao Liu, Guo-Rong Ou, Min-Nian Wang, Tong-Yu Fang, Fu-Huan Chao, Jun-Wen Li.
Study on the resistance of severe acute respiratory syndrome-associated coronavirus
Journal of Virological Methods 126 (2005) 171–177

Haizhou Liu, Vincenzo Naddeo
Removing the novel coronavirus from the water cycle
ScienceDaily, April 3, 2020

DISINFECTING WITH CHLORINE DIOXIDE (CLO$_2$), DST± AND COVALENT SILVER-OZONE

What is Chlorine Dioxide

Chlorine Dioxide (ClO$_2$) is an extremely powerful disinfectant <u>even more effective</u> than Free Chlorine (Cl$_2$) and Sodium Hypochlorite (NaClO). It aggressively kills bacteria, viruses and parasites. ClO$_2$ is widely used across variety of industries, commercial and households as disinfectant, sanitizer and steriliser in foods & beverages processing plants, meat & poultry, hospitals, laboratories, potable drinking water supplies and wastewater treatment plants around the world.

ClO$_2$ presents as a yellowish-green gas that is less toxic and less irritating and has a wider pH range for application. It can be used as both liquid and gas, thus, more environmentally friendly than NaClO.

In 2015, a team of researchers from Osaka University studied the differences between ClO$_2$ and NaClO in anti-bacterial killing efficacy against Multi-Drug Resistant (MDR) bacterial strains such as methicillin-resistant *Staphylococcus aureus* (MRSA) and *Pseudomonas aeruginosa* found Chlorine Dioxide to be <u>far more effective</u> than Sodium Hypochlorite as an anti-bacterial disinfectant.

They found that Chlorine Dioxide whether in 10 ppm or 100 ppm concentrations was able to <u>significantly kill or drastically reduce the numbers of MDR bacteria strains</u> while Sodium Hypochlorite in the same concentrations was only moderately effective (and sometimes not effective) in killing these bacteria strains.

World Health Organization (WHO) – Chlorine Dioxide is WHO approved disinfectant and steriliser in potable drinking water supplies and wastewater treatment plants around the world.

United States Environmental Protection Agency (USEPA) – Chlorine Dioxide is US EPA approved and registered disinfectant, sanitiser and steriliser which is defined as the ability "to destroy or eliminate all forms of microbial including fungi, viruses, and all forms of bacteria and their spores" in food processing plants, potable water supply, hospitals, laboratories and air ventilation systems.

Food and Drug Administration (FDA) – Chlorine Dioxide is FDA approved terminal sanitising rinse on all foods and beverages contact surfaces.

United States Department of Agriculture (USDA) – USDA approval for bacterial and mould control, terminal sanitizing and cleaning in meat and poultry processing plants for environmental surfaces.

Chlorine Dioxide could be one of the most effective sanitizer than Sodium Hypochlorite in disinfection, cleaning and surface protection, especially during this Covid-19 outbreak episode.

Further Advantages of Chlorine Dioxide

- **Wide Applicability.** ClO_2 maintains its disinfecting function over a large pH range while NaClO has a limited range. Also, ClO_2 operates well in temperatures from $5 - 69$ °C while NaClO operates well only under 40 °C.

- **Less affected by interfering factors.** Under clinical settings where biological materials like blood and plasma proteins are present, ClO_2 is able to maintain its disinfecting function while NaClO loses some of its efficacy.

- **Environmentally friendly.** Using ClO_2 as disinfecting agent eliminates formation of toxic halogenated by-products like trihalomethanes (THMs) and chlorinated compounds that are carcinogenic and harmful to the environment.

COVID-19 virus is transmitted during close contact through respiratory droplets (such as through coughing and sneezing). The virus can spread directly from person to person when a COVID-19 case coughs or exhales producing droplets that reach the nose, mouth or eyes of another person. As the droplets are too heavy to be airborne, they land on objects and surfaces surrounding the person. Other people become infected with COVID-19 by touching these contaminated objects or surfaces, then touching their eyes, nose or mouth.

According to the currently available evidence, transmission through smaller droplet nuclei (airborne transmission) that propagate through air at distances longer than 1 meter is limited.

WHO continues to recommend that everyone performs hand hygiene frequently, follows respiratory etiquette recommendations and regularly clean and disinfect surfaces. WHO also continues to recommend the importance of maintaining physical distances and avoiding people with fever or respiratory symptoms. These preventive measures will limit viral transmission.

Why need GoodAire Sanz DST+

GoodAire Sanz DST+ with Nano AgTiO2+ is considered as secondary sanitizing protocol, which is non toxic, non carcinogenic, non corrosive, non tainting, odourless and chemically stable to environmental nature.

In summary, GoodAire Sanz DST+ is:

- Nano Double Silver Titanium Dioxide Plus (DST+) bonds to a treated surface at the molecular level, ensuring that product coatings are not removed by regular routine cleaning processes and traditional detergent solutions. DST+ has proven to neutralize odour-causing microbes on treated surfaces for up to 3 months or longer.

- DST+ is environmentally friendly, non-flammable and have very low toxicity. It contains USEPA (USA's Environmental Protection Agency) approved antimicrobial active ingredients.

- DST+ is specially formulated with ingredient which is non-foaming, non-skin irritating and environmentally friendly. It is made of powerful **COLLOIDAL SILVER, NANO AG+ ION & NANO TiO$_2$** ingredients which offers disinfecting and sanitizing capabilities through its antibacterial, anti-fungicidal and anti-viral properties. DST+ does not contain petroleum distillates, soaps, chemical thickening agents, nitrates, enzymes, phosphates, fatty acids, hydrocarbon toxic solvents, non-biodegradable surfactants and ozone-depleting substances. It doesn't irritate eyes & sensitive skin.

How GoodAire Sanz DST+ Kills Bacteria, Fungi & Virus

GoodAire Sanz DST+ antimicrobial mechanism is based on patented agent's interaction with the microbial cell membrane. It remains chemically active and permanently bond on the treated surface, through a proprietary binding agent. It is durable, non-leaching, non-bleaching, environmentally friendly, effective and safe for the intended applications. Upon contact with microbes, the active compounds of DST+ will penetrate the cell wall and bind into the structure membrane of the microbes. This nano thin film of active layer will disrupt the key functions of the microbes. It will eventually cause the rupture of the cell membrane and kill the microbes.

Inactivation Mechanism of Enveloped Viruses Through GoodAire Sanz DST+

Upon contact with the enveloped viruses, the two active compounds of DST+ namely double nano silver - titanium dioxide (Ag+TiO$_2$) will suppress the virus infectivity through reacting with the viral envelope surface molecules required for binding onto the receptors on the human cells. By interfering with the binding molecules on the virus surface, this results in the loss of ability of the virus to attach to human cells.

What is Goodaire Sanz Covalent Silver-Ozone (DST+O3)

- This covalent silver-ozone hydrosol technology is used by NASA for water purification on the International Space Station - it's the best invention solution that mankind could ever produce.

- For over a hundred years it has been known that oligodynamic of silver ions and ozone gas can mediate extracellular and intracellular immune challenges, due to the oxidation potential of these ions in water.

- Goodaire Sanz's oligodynamic covalent silver ozone hydrosol represents outstanding superb disinfectant properties to modulate disinfect capability and immune events, such as promoting superoxide release and supporting healthy regulation of toxicants.

- Goodaire Sanz's oligodynamic covalent silver ozone hydrosol is one of the most advanced nano-silver [covalently bonded to oxygen] product on the market invented by Mr Richard Yeck, who has impregnated ozone gas into nano silver solution, coupled with titanium dioxide and nano silane coat (DST+).

Human Coronavirus Types

- Coronaviruses are named for the crown-like spikes on their surface. There are four main sub-groupings of coronaviruses, known as alpha, beta, gamma, and delta.

- Human coronaviruses were first identified in the mid-1960s. The seven coronaviruses that can infect people are:

Common human coronaviruses:

- 229E (alpha coronavirus)
- NL63 (alpha coronavirus)
- OC43 (beta coronavirus)
- HKU1 (beta coronavirus)

Other human coronaviruses:

- MERS-CoV (the beta coronavirus that causes Middle East Respiratory Syndrome, or MERS)
- SARS-CoV (the beta coronavirus that causes severe acute respiratory syndrome, or SARS)
- **<u>SARS-CoV-2 (the novel coronavirus that causes coronavirus disease 2019, or COVID-19</u>**
- People around the world commonly get infected with human coronaviruses 229E, NL63, OC43, and HKU1.
- Sometimes coronaviruses that infect animals can evolve and make people sick and become a new human coronavirus. Three recent examples of this are 2019-nCoV, SARS-CoV, and MERS-CoV.

CONCLUSION

GoodAire Sanz DST+ is probably one of the fastest yet most effective disinfectant in the world at 9 seconds killing rate >99.99% and was tested by ALS Technichem, Singapore accredited laboratory.

GoodAire Sanz DST+ was tested to kill human coronavirus i.e. CoV-229E by UNIMAS, Malaysia.

GoodAire Sanz DST+ passed the rabbit eyes and skin exposure test i.e. Sprayed 3 times per day, over 4 weeks period that is not known for immediate and prolong side effects observed by the Guang Dong Detection Center of Microbiology, China.

All the above reports can be provided upon request from GoodAire Pte Ltd, Singapore.

In short, GoodAire Sanz's Chlorine Dioxide, DST+ and Covalent-Silver-TiO2-Ozone are undoubtedly among the very few most advanced disinfectant products in the market.

The inventor, Mr. Richard Yeck has incorporates a *"Total Sanitizing Approach"* via GoodAire Sanz Air Sanitizer system using his proprietary Sanz solutions for **Stage 1 (Chlorine Dioxide), Stage 2 (DST+) and Stage 3 (Covalent-AgTiO2+Ozone)** for the entire terminal disinfection, prevention and protection against COVID-19.

I trust this will keep everyone and every place safe. Let us work together to overcome this challenging period and prevent the spread of COVID-19.

Thank you.

Yours sincerely,

CHANG HEE KUAN *MSc, BSc(Hons), DipBM*